I0421024

The Insulin Resistance Diet

Supercharge Your Energy While Stripping Body-Fat - *Insulin Resistance Diet*

Table of Contents

Contents

Copyright © 2015 by Sage Surefire

All rights reserved. This book or any portion thereof may not be reproduced or used in any manner whatsoever without the express written permission of the publisher except for the use of brief quotations in a book review.

Insulin Resistance Diet Introduction

Imagine doing everything right – eating clean, training hard, taking supplements as advised – and yet still not making any traction on your fat loss goals. Can you imagine how frustrating that would be? Well, chances are if you're reading this you don't need to imagine it – because it is your current reality!

The reason that you are unable to lose body fat likely has more to do with your level of insulin sensitivity than anything else. Insulin sensitivity refers to how much of an insulin response your body gets in response to a given amount of carbohydrate - in other words, how well you body uses blood sugar.

Insulin is one of the most powerful hormones in the body. Its job is to push energy into your muscle, liver and fat cells. Insulin is released from the beta-cells in the pancreatic function of your pancreas. This happens when you take in any type of carbohydrate. How much insulin is released depends on the type of and quantity of carbohydrate that you are consuming. Over training, stress and bad general eating habits can also lead to insulin resistance. Insulin is drawn into the cell by receptor sites on the outside of each cell. If you are over-taxing your pancreas by taking in too many carbs your brain will signal the cells to shut down receptor site function. All of that insulin that should be powering your cells is going to sit around as fat. The key to becoming super lean is to figure out how to become insulin sensitive.

This book will show you exactly how to do just that.

I. Understanding Insulin Resistance

When healthy people eat food, that food that they are eating releases glucose into the blood supply. This glucose in the blood will stimulate a reaction in the pancreas. The pancreas releases a hormone called insulin. Insulin's job is to take the glucose into your muscle cells. This creates ATP for energy, allows you to build muscle and keeps you healthy.

To get the glucose into the muscle cell, it has to first pass through an insulin receptor. The insulin regulator is a bit like a bouncer at a night-club. Insulin is like a VIP guest – it gets an automatic pass. The glucose that it carries with it also gets a free pass.

For people who are insulin resistant, however, it's a whole different story. If the cell is already flushed with glucose, the insulin receptors are not going to allow the insulin to bring any new glycogen in. This can result in an insulin resistance, meaning that, even when it does need the glucose, the cell will be unable to accept it. This increases the level of blood glucose. Yet, the pancreas reads this as a sign that insulin needs to be produced and so just goes on producing more.

So, what happens to all of that excess glucose and insulin. The glucose will be converted into visceral fat – that's the most dangerous sort of fat which surrounds your vital organs. The glucose also gets converted to LDL cholesterol, clogging the arteries and leading to a whole host of cardio pulmonary problems.

How Do You Become Insulin Resistant?

A lot of people are eating way too much nutritionally devoid junk foods that are causing serious problems for their bodies. At the same time, people aren't sleeping properly. They are also far too sedentary. These factors combine to cause insulin sensitivity.

When people eat foods that are high in fructose corn syrup and processed carbohydrates, they are taking huge amounts of glucose into their blood stream. This causes their pancreas to go into overdrive to produce more insulin. This overload of insulin can lead to the insulin receptors that regulate the flow of glucose into the muscle cell shutting down – they no longer do their job. This, in effect, shuts off the muscle cell. It is going to be starved of glucose. It can't make ATP. The muscle cannot get bigger. And the person has no energy.

All of this results from eating the Standard American Diet (SAD).

The super elevated levels of glucose in the blood will lead to . . .

- o Inflammation
- o Fat Gain
- o Memory Loss
- o Fatigue
- o High Blood Pressure
- o Increased Risk of Heart Disease
- o Cirrhosis (liver scarring)
- o Chronic Muscle and Joint Pain
- o Irritable Bowel Syndrome

II. Combatting Insulin Resistance Through Diet

The key to overcoming insulin resistance is diet. The first thing that needs to happen inside your body is normalize your insulin levels. This can only happen one way . . .

By reducing your consumption of sugary, processed carbohydrate foods.

Refined sugar products such as white sugar, candy, sweets and soft drinks, are the biggest culprit in the obesity epidemic that is plaguing the Western world. Added sugar provides absolutely zero essential nutrient quality. As such they are known as empty calories. Sugar is also high in fructose, which can only be broken down by the liver. Too much of it can put overdue stress on your liver, forcing it to turn the fructose into fat and causing fatty liver. Sugar can also cause insulin resistance, which can in turn open the road to diabetes. There is also considerable evidence that too much sugar can contribute to cancer. Sugar, because of its ability to release dopamine in the brain, is highly addictive. And to top it off, sugar will make your teeth rotten.

A Dozen Processed Foods to Ditch Today

- Biscuits
- Crackers
- Pies
- Doughnuts
- Margarine
- Tortilla Chips
- Refined Vegetable Oils
- Soft Drinks
- White Bread
- Pasta
- Bagels

Natural Carbs

Put simply, a natural carb is one that has come out of the ground or off the plant or tree in the form that you are about to eat it. Whole grains come into this category. Even though they are processed to an extent, they retain some of their nutrients and fibers. Processed complex carbs such as pasta, bread and bagels go through an intensive milling, refining and bleaching process that strips away their nutritional value while bulking up the calorie count. You should always opt for wholegrain varieties over processed refined grains.

When you reach for carbs, make sure that they are nutrient dense and that they are low on the glycemic index.

Spotlight on Glycemic Index

The Glycemic Index (GI) is a ranking of carbohydrates from 0 to 100 in accordance with how much they elevate blood sugar levels after food is consumed. High GI foods cause marked fluctuations in blood sugar levels.

Focusing on low GI foods will lower insulin levels as well as insulin resistance.

Fructose has a lower GI than table sugar (sucrose), despite being a lot sweeter.

III. Becoming Sugar Smart

Sweet But Deadly

Sugar is the world's most popular sweetener. It's ascendancy, however, has been relatively recent. Prior to the 18th Century it was a luxury item, available only to the wealthy. In 1700 the average person was eating just 4 pounds of sugar a year. It was only with the opening up of the West Indian and Brazilian sugar cane markets, built on the back of the slave trade, that sugar became affordable to the masses. Today, the average person is eating 4 pounds of sugar every two weeks. During the 'fat is the enemy' era of the 90's, thousands of food products were pumped full of sugar to provide the flavor that was lost when the fat was removed. All of those sugars, however can be categorized 4 ways:

- **Glucose**
- **Galactose**
- **Fructose**
- **Sucrose**

Let's zoom in on them one at a time:

Glucose

During digestion, carbohydrates are broken down into glucose, or blood sugar. These are the body's main source of energy. The glucose is then absorbed into the bloodstream where it is transported to the body's cells. Glucose is the body's main source of energy. Without it, our body and our brain will be unable to function properly.

Glucose is made by plants and stored in the form of sap. Food manufacturers use plant based glucose in the form of such starches as rice, maize, cassava and potatoes to add glucose to their products.

Galactose

Galactose is a type of sugar that provides a compact form of energy in a small package. It is also referred to as 'brain sugar'.

The human body manufactures galactose and it occurs naturally in products such as:

(1)   Dairy Products

(2)   Sugar Beets

(3)   A variety of gums

(4)   Peas

Galactose is not very sweet, so is not a popular alternative to other types of sugar.

Fructose

A simple sugar that is naturally present in foods, fructose is also known as fruit sugar. It gives fruit and other foods their sweet taste. In this natural state, fructose is healthy and safe. The problem occurs when we consume products that have had fructose added to them in the form of high fructose corn-syrup or similar products.

Fructose is metabolized through a different pathway than fructose, namely the liver. During this process uric acid is generated which infiltrates into the cells as well as circulating in the blood. Uric acid is not a friend of your body. In fact, it is toxic. In addition, these fructose added products don't contain the added vitamins to counter the effects of the fructose that would be present in fruits and vegetables.

In addition to building up uric acid, fructose will also:

- Increase triglycerides, which stimulate mid-section fat deposits

- Stimulate your appetite

- Increase your LDL (bad) fat levels

- Increase blood pressure

- Increase your risk of heart disease

- Increase the risk of gout

In addition, drinking fruit juice provides fructose without the addition of vitamins and antioxidants.

Sucrose

When glucose and fructose combine we get sucrose. The sucrose that proliferates in most household kitchens today has been processed. The consumption of sucrose has exploded since the 1970's. It's no surprise that this has been mirrored by an equally explosive obesity epidemic. Over that same 50 years a host of artificial sweeteners have also emerged onto the marketplace. These include:

o High fructose corn syrup

o Saccharin

o Sucralose

o Aspartame

o Cyclamate

o Stevia

Sugar is a great food preservative, which is one reason why it gets added to virtually every type of food you can possibly imagine. Combine that with the proven, scientific fact that sugar is more addictive than cocaine and it's little wonder that were all drowning in a cesspool of obesity and its associated problems. Because sugar is in everything, we often don't even realize when we're consuming it. That's what we call hidden sugars. Here are some common items that contain alarming levels of hidden sucrose:

• Soup

• Ketchup

• Canned vegetables

• "Low Fat" products

- Fruit Yogurt

- Chinese Takeaways

- Soda

- Dried Fruit

- Granola Bars

- Energy Drinks

Energy drinks, fruit juices and sodas attack your body on two fronts as the combined effects of glucose and fructose play havoc with your system. Your blood sugar levels will get an immediate spike from the glucose. In response to this, the pancreas will elevate its insulin manufacture. The fructose in your drink will fast track it to your liver, where it is converted into fat, with the by- products of triglycerides and uric acid. Meanwhile, the excess amount of insulin in your system will stimulate your appetite. Now, remember that all of this has resulted from a liquid – you haven't eaten anything. Yet, you now have a craving to do just that. You reach for something sweet – and the whole destructive process is replicated.

That's why energy drinks, sodas and fruit juices don't belong in your life. Make the smarter choice and consume natural fruits and vegetables, which come ready packed with vitamins, minerals, amino acids and anti-oxidants. The bottom line on sucrose is that it is dangerous. Yet there is no benefit to that risk. It gets added to your food simply to get it past your taste buds. It has absolutely no nutritional value to you. You need to get it under control. How? Simply by making smarter choices. Of course, that's not easy. Sugar, after all, is big business. It's also addictive. And it's everywhere. You will never completely eliminate sugar from your diet. But you can become it's master, rather than it's slave, which is the case with the majority of the people around you.

Becoming Sugar Aware

In order to gain mastery over sugar, you need to learn to observe how your body reacts to this sweet poison. Becoming sugar aware involves:

- *Reading the labels* - Become aware of the various names for sugar. Keep aware of the fact that the nearer an item is to the top of the list, the more of it there is in the product.

- *Knowing what everyday foods you eat that are sugar loaded.*

- *Observing how your body reacts to sugar, especially fructose and high fructose corn syrup.*

- *Monitoring how you feel upon waking* – do you feel like springing out of bed or like rolling over and going back to sleep?

- *Monitoring your sense of taste and smell .*

- *Checking the color of your urine* – the lighter the better!

- *Getting a journal and recording your observations regarding sugar and how your body reacts to it.*

- *Going through your pantry and separating all the foods that contain an unhealthy level of sugar.* Mark these items with colored tape.

- *Making a list of all the artificial sweeteners that you use.* Mark these with another colored tape. If it contains both sugar and artificial sweeteners put both pieces of tape on it.

- *Recruiting the other members of your family to support you in your quest to gain mastery over sugar.*

Artificial White Death

With the myriad problems associated with sugar, taking an artificial sweetener to get your daily fix may seem like a good idea. What you may not realize is that many of those sugar substitutes can actually be hazardous to your health. So, why are artificial sweeteners so bad for us?

The key is in the very name. Anything labeled artificial is usually created by a chemist in a laboratory. The resultant product cannot be easily digested by the body, In fact, study after study links these chemicals to imbalances created inside the body. This research has linked artificial sweeteners to:

- Depression

- Joint aches

- Alzheimer's disease

- Parkinson's disease

- Cancer

- Death

Furthermore, there is no concrete evidence to show that these sugar substitutes even help people to lose weight. On the contrary, studies show that chemical sweeteners actually stimulate the appetite and lead to obesity. Let's take a closer look at the common artificial sweeteners you're likely to run across.

Sucralose

Sucralose is made from real sugar that is chemically modified to be calorie-free. They do this by adding chlorine. But that's not all. Other chemicals used in the manufacture of sucralose are acetone (a key ingredient of nail-polish remover), benzene (an ingredient used in oil and gasoline), methanol (used in windshield washer fluid) and formaldehyde (used to preserve dead bodies). Some of the chemicals used to make sucralose are listed on the US Environmental Protection Agency's list of most deadly poisons.

Aspartame

Aspartame is sometimes listed on food labels as phenylalanine. It has been the subject of a lot of heated controversy, both because of both safety issues and questionable circumstances surrounding it's FDA approval. Aspartame is the cause of more complaints to the FDA than any other food. Aspartame use can lead to:

• Memory loss

• Headaches

• Dizziness

• Seizures

• Nausea

• Weight Gain

• Depression

• Insomnia

• Fatigue

This is just a partial list. Aspartame has 92 official side-effects that have been reported to the FDA. One of them is Parkinson's Disease. In fact, many people believe that it was his constant exposure to Aspartame as a result of his endorsement of Diet Pepsi that led to Michael J. Fox's developing Parkinson's Disease at the unprecedented age of 29 years. Still, Aspartame is used in over 6,000 products worldwide. These include:

o Sodas

o Cereals

o Chewing Gum

o Desserts

o Breath mints

o Teas

o Coffees

o Yogurt

Saccharine

Throughout the 1960's and '70's studies showed that saccharine was linked to Cancer in animals. In 1977, the FDA proposed a ban on this sugar substitute, but had to be satisfied with a warning label on the packet. Saccharine is a coal-tar derivative and has absolutely no food value. It is created by chemists in a laboratory.

One of the chemicals used to create saccharin is ammonia, which is also used for cleaning toilets. Other chemicals used to make saccharine are sulphur dioxide and chlorine. Common side-effects are headaches, diarrhea and itching hives. By the year 2001, 30 more studies had been conducted which showed that saccharin does not cause cancer in adults.

Saccharine is often used to sweeten drinks. This causes even more problems for your body. When you gulp down your saccharine sweetened soda, the pancreas responds by upping insulin production. In effect, your body is expecting food and getting prepared to digest it. But, unless you eat something with your soda, no food will accompany the liquid that has just gone down your throat. This will lead to a craving for high carb food in order to allow the insulin to do their job. That's why saccharine has been linked to weight gain and obesity.

Acesulflame K

This sweetener is 200 times sweeter than sucrose. It is made by chlorinating sugar. It has a negative impact on the thyroid. When your thyroid isn't working well, your metabolism is affected and you are not burning as many calories. One in five Americans are on thyroid medication, many of them as a result of their addiction to diet sodas that contain Acesulflame K. In 1988 Acesuflame K was listed as a potential substance that causes cancer by the Center for Science in the Public Interest after a number of studies showed a direct relation to the growth of tumors and leukemia in animals.

Agave

Agave contains calories, unlike the sweeteners mentioned above. Agave nectar is a natural sweetener produced from the agave plant. The juice is extracted from the plant's core, filtered, heated, treated with enzymes and then concentrated until it becomes a syrupy liquid.

The main problem with agave nectar is that it contains high levels of fructose. Studies have shown that high amounts of fructose in the body can promote triglyceride levels. High triglycerides are a known risk factor for heart disease. Eating fructose can also cause bloating, gas and stomach discomfort. In addition, fructose is bad news for your liver.

High Fructose Corn Syrup (HFCS)

High fructose corn syrup is the most abundant sugar. The average American consumes about 70 pounds of it each year. In high fructose corn syrup, fructose and glucose are not chemically attached. The fructose is immediately delivered to your liver. It turns on a fat production mechanism that can lead to fatty liver. It can also lead to:

• Heart disease

• Cancer

• Dementia

• Diabetes

There are also chemical contaminants in high fructose corn syrup. These include chloralkali, which contains mercury. With the average person consuming some 20 teaspoons a day of high fructose corn syrup, this can lead to a deadly build-up of mercury in your system.

High fructose corn syrup is a signal that the food which contains it is low quality. It will be processed and full of toxins that will destroy your health. You need to go into your kitchen and identify the foods that contain HFCS. Collect them all up in your arms and drop them into the garbage bin.

White Bread

That loaf of bread that looks so appetizing is, in fact, a gooey, indigestible and incomplete protein, a few multivitamins and a whole lot of sugar. White bread, in particular, is problematic to the body. It's empty calories, bleached flour and has all the nutrients stripped out of it. That's why most health conscious people tend to go with whole wheat bread. Recently, sprouted grain bread, not made with flour, has also become popular. Sprouted grain bread contains real, living grains with all the nutrients and fiber retained.

IV. Foods That Reverse Insulin Resistance

While food is a big part of the insulin resistance problem, it is also part of the solution. The following foods have been proven to improve insulin sensitivity.

Avocado

The soluble fiber in the avocado stabilizes blood sugar and lowers cholesterol. It, thus, helps fight insulin resistance. The healthy mono-saturated fats in avocados also help the body to better absorb anti-cancer antioxidants. The plant sterols in the avocado also have been shown to lower cholesterol.

Cinnamon

Cinnamon is a common spice that is available everywhere. It comes from inside bark of the cinnamonomum plant and is a rich source of natural antioxidants. Researchers have studied the effect of cinnamon on people with both type 1 and type 2 diabetes, and have also researched the effect it has on the blood sugar of people without diabetes. The spice Cinnamon contains a compound known as cinnamaldehyde. This compound has been shown to reduced blood sugar levels and increase pancreatic production of insulin.

Eggs

Eggs are an ideal source of protein. They are also extremely low in sugar count. This makes them an ideal food to improve insulin resistance. Eggs are a cheap form of a whole host of health giving nutrients. They are an ideal base to build your breakfast upon.

Sweet Potatoes

Sweet potatoes, despite their name, do not contain many sugars. They contain an enzyme which converts most of its starches into sugars as the potato matures. They also contain a large amount of carotenoids, which are orange and yellow pigments that play a role in helping the body respond to insulin. In addition, they are rich in chlorogenic acid, which is also believed to reduce insulin resistance.

Fiber

Fiber is what gives shape and stability to plants. It's the indigestible part of the plant, as opposed to starch, which is the form of energy in plants. Fiber passes through the digestive tract without all the calorie energy being absorbed. Fiber provides bulk to the intestinal contents, promotes healthy digestion and elimination, improves digestion and wards off all types of cancer.

Fiber can be separated into soluble and insoluble varieties. Most plants contain both types but vary in their ratio.

- o Soluble fiber dissolves in water

- o Insoluble fiber does not dissolve in water

Soluble fiber has been shown to lower your blood sugar and LDL cholesterol. Insoluble fiber helps prevent constipation by helping to form bulk in your stools. Here are 8 more benefits of increasing your fiber intake:

- It decreases stress on the liver

- It promotes intestinal bacteria

- It decreases cancer-causing toxins

- It contains anti-oxidants that protect from liver damage

- It contains chlorophyll which prevents the gut from absorbing toxins

- It helps to treat non-alcoholic fatty liver disease

- It assists in the removal of LDL (bad) cholesterol

- It lowers triglyceride levels

Legumes are a special type of fiber, which are also high in protein. They are the seeds of plants. Legumes contain phytic acid, which have been shown to protect us from liver and colon cancer. The following legumes should be part of your weekly eating plan:

- Beans

- Peas

- Peanuts

- Lentils

- Alfalfa

Fiber in Fruit

Most fruits are high in both fiber and fructose. We've already learnt that fructose can cause problems to the body and, when the natural casing is taken away, fructose can be toxic. When you eat whole fruit, though, the negative impact of the fructose is negated by fiber. That's why an orange is a whole lot healthier than a glass of orange juice.

Canned fruits are even worse than fruit juices. The canning process not only breaks down the fiber, it also robs the fruit of most of its nutrients. Anything in a can is best avoided.

Peeling vegetables and fruits can also remove much of their health benefits. However, if a vegetable or fruit contains a pip, it doesn't need peeling. Make sure though, that all fruits and vegetables are thoroughly washed before consuming.

Grains

Many people are confused about grains. As a result of theirfavored position at the base of the "food pyramid" many people think that they are good for you, that they provide essential fiber and that they are low in fat. The reality is that they are none of those things. Not only are they unhealthy, they are actually toxic to the body. Pasta, bread, bagels and cereal are all processed grains. Milling, refining and bleaching the grains decreases their nutritional value while increasing the calorie's density. Whole grain varieties are better because they retain some of the nutrients and fiber, but even these are somewhat processed and may be high in calories.

From now on, eat only whole grains. That means:

- No white rice

- No white flour

- No white pasta

Be careful when buying bread. It may look like whole wheat but could simply be white bread with artificial coloring added. Check the label. If it doesn't say "100% whole wheat", put it back on the shelf.

V. Shopping Tips

Follow these tips to ensure that your pantry and refrigerator are always stocked with safe, healthy, delicious food options:

- o Buy fresh organic food whenever possible

- o Use Farmer's Markets to buy locally

- o Only purchase organic poultry, fish and eggs

- o Only buy organic versions of the following:

- o Apples

- o Celery

- o Cherry Tomatoes

- o Cucumbers

- o Grapes

- o Nectarines

- o Peaches

- o Potatoes

- o Snap Peas

- o Spinach

- o Strawberries

- o Sweet Bell Peppers

- Hot Peppers

- Kale

- Collards

- Make sure that organic foods purchased are labeled "certified organically grown."

- Shop only on the outside aisles of the grocery store

- Don't buy anything that would last more than 3 days on your counter

VI. Sample Recipes

Breakfast

It is really important that you eat a real, healthy breakfast. The heartier the first meal of the day is, the better. A decent breakfast will allow you to fire up your metabolism and get your hunger under control for the coming day.

Want to know how important eating breakfast is? A landmark study by the US National Weight Control Registry (NWCR) identified that, of members who had lost an average of 66 pounds and kept it off for 5 years, 90% of them ate breakfast on most days of the week. Breakfast eaters also reported higher levels of physical activity. In contrast, breakfast skippers tended to make poor food choices. Don't be one of them; make it your routine every day to have a nutritious breakfast so that you're well fuelled and mentally sharp for the day ahead.

Almond Flour Coconut Waffles

Serves: 1-2

Ingredients

- o 1.5 cup almond flour/meal
- o 2 eggs, whisked
- o 1/4 cup canned coconut milk 1/4 cup unsweetened shredded coconut
- o 1 tablespoon arrowroot powder or coconut flour 1 tablespoon raw honey
- o 1 teaspoon vanilla extract 1/2 teaspoon baking soda
- o 1/2 teaspoon sea salt
- o 1/2 teaspoon cinnamon

Instructions

- ➤ Whisk your eggs in a medium-large sized bowl. Add your coconut milk and whisk together with eggs Next add your almond flour and mix together
- ➤ Add your shredded coconut, arrowroot powder, baking soda and mix together
- ➤ Lastly, add in your honey, vanilla, salt and cinnamon Mix together thoroughly. Pour into your waffle iron and heat until cooked through.

Poached Eggs In Avocado

Serves 2

(What a fantastic breakfast, lunch, snack idea! Packed with protein, essential fatty acids and loads of minerals!)

Ingredients

- o 3 Eggs

- o 3 Avocados

Instructions

- ➤ Poach eggs according to your tastes and then simply place them in avocado and sprinkle with pepper.

Vegetable Soup

Serves 2

Ingredients

- Green Beans
- Celery
- Zucchini
- Yellow Squash
- Red Peppers
- Leeks
- Onions
- Garlic
- Shredded Cabbage
- Vegetable Broth
- Oregano
- Basil
- Salt

Instructions

- Cut up and combine vegetables in a pot of heated vegetable broth.
- Bring to the boil and then simmer for 15 minutes.
- Add salt, oregano and basil for flavor.
- Serve with sprouted wheat tortillas that have been lightly toasted.

Lunch

Lunch can be a tricky meal. Often we're not at home when we eat it. But, whether you're eating at home, the office, or on the go, what you put in your mouth at midday can either keep your metabolism humming or send you spiraling toward mid-afternoon cravings. Here are 6 key tips to allow you to make smart lunch choices . . .

(1) Pack in Protein

(2) Use dark greens as a salad base

(3) Add color to your salads

(4) Fill up on fiber

(5) Go with smoothies (add frozen fruit)

(6) Use Greek Yoghurt for flavor

Easy Guacamole Salad

Serves 3-4

Ingredients

- 3 small avocados chopped
- 1 large ripe but firm tomato chopped
- 1 small green chili chopped
- 1 can black beans
- 1/2 small onion chopped
- 1/2 tsp freshly grated lime zest
- 25 grams of coriander chopped
- 2 tablespoons of lemon or lime juice
- 1 pinch of Celtic sea salt
- 1/4 tsp ground cayenne pepper
- 1/s tsp minced garlic

Instructions

- Place the tomato, green chili, black beans, onion and lime zest into a large bowl
- Whisk together the lime juice, olive oil, sea salt, garlic and cayenne pepper over the vegetables. Toss well
- Just before serving fold the avocado into the salad. Check the seasoning and serve at room temperature.

Frittata Bites

(Frittata bites are handy to have as they keep up to 3 days in a Tupperware container in the fridge)

Serves 3-4

Ingredients

- o 4 eggs
- o 1/2 cup of goats feta
- o 1/2 cup almond milk
- o 1 small zucchini finely grated
- o 1/3 cup of semi dried tomatoes
- o 2 green spring onions finely chopped

Instructions

- ➢ Heat over to 180 degrees Celsius Grease a 12 hole muffin pan
- ➢ In a bowl, whisk eggs, feta, and almond milk (I then season with herbs from my garden!)
- ➢ Combine remaining ingredients in the mix above
- ➢ Pour into muffin pan and bake for 20-25 minutes until brown and firm...place in your lunch box with a salad!

Salmon & Tuna Muffins With Lime Dipping Sauce

High in protein and essential fatty acids, these tasty muffins will keep you going through the day without having that 3pm lull. They're easy to make and if you make them over the weekend you have them to enjoy for lunch or as a snack throughout the week.

Serves 2-3

Ingredients

- o 3 Cloves Of Garlic Crushed
- o 2 Teaspoons Of Sesame Oil
- o 1 Teaspoon Of Chopped Lemongrass
- o 1 Tablespoon Of Chopped Ginger
- o 1 Egg Beaten
- o 2 Tablespoons Of Chopped Coriander
- o 425g Tin Of Tuna Or Salmon
- o 1 Tsp Of Red Chili(Optional)

Dipping Sauce

- o 1/2 Cup Rice Wine
- o Vinegar
- o 2 Tablespoons Of Lime Juice
- o 1 Large Red Chili
- o A Tablespoon Of Coriander

Instructions

- ➤ Preheat oven to 180 degrees c. Line mini muffin tray.

- ➤ Place all ingredients for the muffin into a food processor until well combined.

- ➤ Spoon mixture into muffin holes and bake for 10 minutes or until cooked through.

- ➤ For the dipping sauce place all ingredients into a bowl and mix well.

- ➤ Serve with fish cakes and a nice salad.

Dinner

In the Western world we don't do dinner very well. We generally eat way too much, and not enough of the right stuff. In fact, a survey of the healthiness of the food revealed that the goodness of what we eat decreases 1.7 percent for every hour that passes in the day. Other research reports that dinner is 15.9 percent less healthy than breakfast on average. This section gives you the power to hit those statistics for six.

Coconut Chicken Or Fish

Serves 4

SERVED WITH SPINACH/AVOCADO/MANGO AND BLUEBERRY SALAD SPRINKLED WITH PEPITAS

Ingredients

- o 1 450 ml can of coconut milk
- o 4 pieces of chicken or fish of your choice
- o 1/2 cup lime juice
- o 1 tsp curry powder

Instructions

- ➢ In the morning take four pieces of chicken or fish and soak in a can of coconut milk with half a cup of lime juice and a teaspoon of curry powder.
- ➢ In the evening grill your chicken or fish.

Salad

> Combine spinach, half a mango, a full pun net of blueberries and a full avocado...

Tuna Salad

Serves 4

Walnuts will dress up your tuna salad. It's tastier when the walnuts are toasted. Walnuts are great for your brain function.

Ingredients

o 1 can tuna in olive oil

o 1 large stalk celery, chopped

o 1 small cucumber, sliced

o 1/4 cup chopped walnuts

o 1 small tomato chopped

o 1 cup of spinach

o Season to taste

Instructions

> Combine all the ingredients in a bowl except the spinach.

> Drizzle with dressing of your choice, season with fresh herbs.

> Place on spinach leaves over your plate and enjoy!

Salmon, Feta & Pumpkin Pie

Serves 4

Ingredients

- o 6 eggs
- o Butter
- o Spring onions
- o A good handful of Blanched spinach (drained and dried off in kitchen towel)
- o Garlic Pumpkin slices just steamed slightly to be soft to eat Feta & Almond meal (a good shake)

Instructions

- ➢ Preheat oven to 180c
- ➢ Pan fry spring onions garlic and butter/oil Blanch spinach and dry well.
- ➢ Steam pumpkin so it's soft enough to eat. Place eggs, spring onion mix, almond meal, crumbled feta in a big bowl andmix.
- ➢ Place almond pastry if using this into the bottom of a deep oven dish.
- ➢ Layer some (not much) of the mixed ingredients on bottom and Squash down firmly.
- ➢ Next layer put smoked salmon (Huon cold smoked pieces available In deli $6.99) or fresh Smoked pieces.. thinner and more expensive) then add pumpkin slices, then add the remaining liquid mix...
- ➢ Place in the oven for 30-40 minutes or until browned.

It can be eaten warm or cold and keeps in the fridge a few days.

Sage Surefire

Subscribe to our list to get notified of new book releases from Sage Surefire. We notify you of new book releases, updates to the books, and when a book is given away free.

Click here to subscribe

You'll like my other books.

Women Bodybuilding: Build a lean, sexy, toned, curvy body without getting bulky

http://www.amazon.com/gp/product/B00YB9SAN0?*Version*=1&*entries*=0

CrossFit Training: Build a lean, athletic, sexy body with fresh and exciting crossfit workouts

http://www.amazon.com/gp/product/B00Z14BENW?*Version*=1&*entries*=0

Building Muscle: Bullshit free secrets to building muscle

http://www.amazon.com/gp/product/B010INJBPS?*Version*=1&*entries*=0

HIIT Workouts: Get HIIT fit, fast-track your way to a shredded, super-fit new you

http://www.amazon.com/gp/product/B010MSYK96?*Version*=1&*entries*=0

Absolute Fitness Kettlebell Workouts

http://www.amazon.com/gp/product/B010Z9TJDO

Resistance Training: Tone Your Body For A Lifetime Of Great Health

http://www.amazon.com/gp/product/B011SDRLZY

www.ingramcontent.com/pod-product-compliance
Lightning Source LLC
Chambersburg PA
CBHW070449290526
45791CB00005B/2106